Fast Like a Girl

Concise

A Woman's Guide to Using the Healing Power of Fasting to Burn Fat, Boost Energy, and Balance Hormones

(Pelz Collection)

Author

Julia W. Boehm, Mindy Pelz

Copyright © 2023, All Rights Reserved.

Publisher's Note

This document provides accurate and reliable information on the subject. Because the publisher is not required to provide accounting, licensed, or qualified services, the publication is sold. Order a legal or professional expert for advice.

Copying, printing, or transmitting this document is illegal. Recording and storing this publication without written permission from the publisher is prohibited. Rights reserved.

The reader is solely responsible for any liability resulting from using or abusing policies, processes, or directions in this document.

The publisher is not liable for any damages, losses, or reparations caused by the information herein.

Copyright © 2023 Julia W. Boehm and Mindy Pelz

Copyright fuels creativity, encourages diverse voices, promotes free speech, and creates a vibrant culture. Thank you for buying a copy of this book.

A portion of this work first appeared in The Utne Reader and Fast Like a Girl.

Note to Readers.

Note that this book is concise with different experiences about life with easy understanding.

ISBN: 978-1-312-25264-6

Contents

Introduction 1
   Welcome to the World of Fasting 1
   The Female Body and Fasting 3
Part I 6
Understanding Fasting 6
   What is Fasting and How Does It Work? 6
   Benefits of Fasting 8
   Debunking Fasting Myths and Misconceptions 10
Part II 13
The Science Behind Female Fasting 13
   The Physiology of Women and Fasting 13
   Hormones and Fasting 15
   How Fasting Impacts Female Metabolism 17
Part III 20
Preparing for a Successful Fast 20
   Setting Your Intention 20
   Creating a Safe and Effective Fasting Plan 22
   Overcoming Common Challenges in Female Fasting 24
Part IV 27
Fasting for Weight Loss and Fat Burning 27
   Fasting for Weight Loss 27
   The Role of Autophagy in Fat Burning 29
   Combining Fasting with Exercise for Optimal Results 30
Part V 33
Fasting for Energy and Performance 33

- Harnessing the Power of Fasting for Increased Energy Levels 33
- Fasting for Physical and Mental Performance 35
- Fasting for Improved Athletic Performance 36

Part VI 38

Fasting for Hormonal Balance 38
- The Impact of Fasting on Hormonal Health 38
- Fasting to Regulate Menstrual Cycles and PMS Symptoms 40
- Managing Menopause and Hormonal Changes through Fasting 42

Part VII 45

Integrating Fasting into Your Lifestyle 45
- Building a Sustainable Fasting Routine 45
- Combining Fasting with Other Dietary Approaches 47
- Navigating Social Situations and Maintaining Fasting Consistency 49

Conclusion 52
- Embracing the Journey of Fasting 52

Appendix 54
- A. Sample Fasting Plans and Protocols 54
- B. Fasting-Friendly Recipes and Meal Ideas 54

Introduction

Welcome to the World of Fasting

In an era where health and wellness take center stage, the ancient practice of fasting has emerged as a powerful tool for enhancing physical, mental, and emotional well-being. Welcome to the world of fasting, a realm where millennia-old traditions and cutting-edge science converge to offer women a path to burn fat, boost energy, and balance hormones. This journey towards self-discovery and empowerment is marked by profound insights into the body's inherent ability to heal and rejuvenate through deliberate abstention from food.

Fasting, as an integral aspect of human history, has been practiced across cultures and religions for various reasons, ranging from spiritual purification to physical cleansing. However, it is only in recent times that the medical and scientific communities have delved deeper into the potential health benefits of fasting. As women's health and wellness have gained prominence in research, the unique and intricate relationship between fasting and the female body has come to light, captivating the attention of scholars, practitioners, and health enthusiasts alike.

The world of fasting welcomes women to a realm of self-discovery, where understanding the physiological intricacies of the female body becomes paramount. Women's bodies, with their cyclical hormonal fluctuations and distinct metabolic responses, present a fascinating tapestry of complexities that necessitate tailored approaches to fasting. Here, in this immersive exploration, the healing potential of fasting takes center stage, illuminating how women can optimize their well-being, seize their health journey, and foster a deeper connection with their bodies.

Within these pages, we embark on a voyage to unravel the science behind female fasting, discerning how the body responds to periods of nourishment restriction and how hormones play an indispensable role in this dynamic interplay. From the intricacies of autophagy, the cellular self-cleansing process, to the profound impact of fasting on hormonal balance, every chapter endeavors to illuminate the transformative effects of fasting on a woman's physical and emotional landscape.

As women take their first steps into the world of fasting, they are met with empowering insights into the preparation and planning necessary for a successful fasting journey. Setting intentions, designing personalized fasting regimens, and surmounting common challenges become essential components of this expedition toward health optimization. Armed with knowledge and determination, women can confidently embrace fasting as a holistic lifestyle approach, catering to their individual needs and priorities.

The world of fasting welcomes women to embrace fasting not merely as a means of temporary weight loss but as a sustainable and gratifying practice, enhancing energy levels, mental clarity, and athletic performance. Integrating fasting into daily life, forging a harmonious relationship with food, and navigating social situations become the cornerstones of lasting success on this transformative path.

As we traverse through this comprehensive guide, "Fast Like a Girl: A Woman's Guide to Using the Healing Power of Fasting to Burn Fat, Boost Energy, and Balance Hormones," readers will find themselves equipped with invaluable knowledge, evidence-based strategies, and practical tips to harness the healing potential of fasting. Empowering women to reclaim agency over their health, this book endeavors to serve as a lifelong companion, supporting individuals on their journey towards holistic well-being and a deeper appreciation for the body's inherent wisdom.

Welcome to the world of fasting—a realm where women can tap into their inner strength, embrace their uniqueness, and unlock the transformative power of fasting to cultivate a healthier, happier, and more vibrant life. The adventure awaits, and with it comes the promise of a rejuvenated body, a reinvigorated spirit, and a profound sense of self-discovery. Let us embark on this voyage together, celebrating the extraordinary capabilities of the female body and the boundless possibilities that fasting unveils for those willing to embrace its transformative embrace.

The Female Body and Fasting

Fasting, a practice with deep historical roots, has garnered significant attention in recent years for its potential health benefits. However, as women step into the world of fasting, they encounter a unique and intricate relationship between their bodies and this age-old tradition. "The Female Body and Fasting: Unraveling the Connection" delves into the physiological complexities that underpin fasting for women, shedding light on the dynamic interplay between the female body and this transformative practice.

Women's bodies are finely tuned instruments, orchestrating a symphony of hormonal fluctuations and metabolic processes throughout their menstrual cycles and beyond. The distinct nature of these physiological rhythms necessitates a nuanced approach to fasting—one that recognizes and honors the intricacies of the female body.

At the heart of this exploration lies an understanding of how fasting affects the female body's delicate hormonal balance. Hormones, the messengers of the body, regulate a myriad of functions, from metabolism and energy regulation to mood and reproduction. Fasting, when implemented mindfully, can positively influence hormone levels, fostering a sense of balance and harmony within the female body.

One of the key focal points in "The Female Body and Fasting: Unraveling the Connection" is the impact of fasting on the menstrual cycle and reproductive health. Delving into scientific research and expert insights, this chapter elucidates the potential effects of fasting on menstruation, fertility, and hormonal disorders. Understanding these ramifications empowers women to make informed choices about fasting that align with their individual health needs and goals.

As we continue to unravel the connection between the female body and fasting, we explore the metabolic responses that differ between men and women during fasting periods. Research suggests that women may experience unique metabolic adaptations to fasting, further emphasizing the importance of tailoring fasting protocols to suit female physiology.

Beyond hormonal and metabolic aspects, this chapter addresses the psychological and emotional dimensions of fasting for women. Mindful fasting practices can lead to enhanced emotional resilience and an improved relationship with food and body image. By cultivating a compassionate and intuitive approach to fasting, women can foster a deeper connection with their bodies and embark on a journey of self-discovery.

"The Relationship Between the Female Body and Fasting: Understanding the Connection" aims to provide women with the necessary information and insights to engage in fasting practices while honoring and appreciating their bodies' inherent wisdom. By acknowledging the intricacies of the female physiology and its distinct reactions to fasting, women have the opportunity to utilize this transformative practice as a potent means of enhancing their overall health, well-being, and sense of empowerment.

In this chapter, we cordially invite readers to embrace the practice of fasting as a customized and adaptable approach that acknowledges and respects the unique characteristics of the female body. With a thorough comprehension of the physiological dynamics involved, women can adeptly navigate the realm of fasting and harness its therapeutic capabilities to optimize their well-being, promote hormonal equilibrium, and unlock their utmost potential. "The Relationship Between the Female Body and Fasting: Exploring the Connection" establishes the foundation for a profound exploration, highlighting the endurance, power, and insight of the female body as it embarks on a journey towards comprehensive wellness and personal enlightenment.

Part I

Understanding Fasting

What is Fasting and How Does It Work?

Fasting is a practice of voluntarily abstaining from food and, in some cases, certain beverages for a specific period. It is an ancient tradition that has been practiced for various reasons, including spiritual, cultural, and health purposes. In recent years, fasting has gained significant attention in the health and wellness community due to emerging scientific research supporting its potential benefits.

How Fasting Works:

1. Metabolic Switch: When we consume food, our bodies use the carbohydrates from the meal as the primary source of energy. During fasting, as the body depletes its carbohydrate stores, it undergoes a metabolic switch and starts utilizing stored fats for energy. This process is called ketosis, and it is a central mechanism in several fasting protocols.

2. Hormonal Changes: Fasting triggers several hormonal changes in the body. The most well-known is the increase in human growth hormone (HGH), which supports fat metabolism, muscle gain, and overall cellular repair. Additionally, fasting can lead to lower insulin levels, promoting fat burning and reducing the risk of insulin resistance.

3. Autophagy: Fasting induces a process called autophagy, where the body starts to break down and recycle damaged cellular components. This cellular self-cleaning mechanism

plays a crucial role in maintaining cellular health and has been linked to longevity and disease prevention.

4. Caloric Deficit: Fasting naturally creates a caloric deficit since no calories are consumed during the fasting period. This can lead to weight loss over time, assuming that the individual does not compensate by overeating during non-fasting periods.

5. Improved Insulin Sensitivity: Regular fasting has been shown to improve insulin sensitivity, which is crucial for maintaining stable blood sugar levels and reducing the risk of type 2 diabetes.

Types of Fasting:

There are various fasting approaches, and each has its unique structure and benefits. Some popular types of fasting include:

1. Intermittent Fasting (IF): Involves cycling between periods of eating and fasting. Common methods include the 16/8 method (fasting for 16 hours, eating within an 8-hour window) or the 5:2 method (eating normally for 5 days, and significantly reducing calorie intake on 2 non-consecutive days).

2. Alternate-Day Fasting: This method involves alternating between fasting days (with very minimal calorie intake) and regular eating days.

3. Extended Fasting: Longer fasting periods that may last 24 hours, 48 hours, or even several days. Extended fasting typically requires medical supervision and is not recommended for everyone.

4. Time-Restricted Eating: Similar to intermittent fasting, this approach restricts eating to specific hours of the day, but it might not involve complete fasting during the non-eating hours.

It is essential to note that fasting may not be suitable for everyone, and individual experiences can vary. Pregnant or breastfeeding women, individuals with certain medical conditions, and those with a history of disordered eating should approach fasting with caution or seek guidance from a healthcare professional.

Ultimately, understanding the mechanisms and different types of fasting can help individuals make informed decisions about incorporating fasting into their lifestyle and exploring its potential benefits on health and well-being. Before starting any fasting regimen, it is advisable to consult with a healthcare provider to ensure it aligns with individual health needs and goals.

Benefits of Fasting

Fasting offers a range of potential benefits, both for physical health and overall well-being. It is important to note that individual experiences may vary, and the benefits of fasting may depend on factors such as the fasting method, individual health status, and adherence to a balanced diet during non-fasting periods. Some of the potential benefits of fasting include:

1. Weight Loss: Fasting can lead to a caloric deficit, promoting weight loss over time. When done correctly, fasting may help reduce body fat while preserving lean muscle mass.

2. Improved Insulin Sensitivity: Fasting has been shown to improve insulin sensitivity, helping to regulate blood sugar levels and reduce the risk of type 2 diabetes.

3. Enhanced Fat Burning: During fasting, the body enters a state of ketosis, where it uses stored fats for energy, leading to increased fat burning.

4. Autophagy and Cellular Repair: Fasting triggers autophagy, a process where the body removes damaged cells and components, promoting cellular repair and renewal.

5. Cardiovascular Health: Fasting has been associated with improvements in various cardiovascular risk factors, such as reduced blood pressure, lower cholesterol levels, and decreased triglycerides.

6. Brain Health and Mental Clarity: Some studies suggest that fasting may have neuroprotective effects, supporting brain health and enhancing cognitive function.

7. Reduced Inflammation: Fasting may help reduce chronic inflammation, which is linked to various health conditions, including autoimmune diseases.

8. Increased Human Growth Hormone (HGH) Levels: Fasting can elevate HGH levels, which play a role in fat metabolism, muscle gain, and overall cellular repair.

9. Longevity: Some animal studies indicate that intermittent fasting may extend lifespan, although further research is needed to confirm its effects on human longevity.

10. Immune System Support: Fasting may enhance the immune system's response, as it allows the body to allocate resources to repair and protect against potential threats.

11. Psychological Benefits: Fasting can promote mindfulness and improve the relationship with food, leading to a better understanding of hunger cues and eating habits.

12. Gut Health: Fasting may positively influence gut microbiota, supporting a healthy gut environment and digestive function.

It is important to approach fasting mindfully and consider individual health conditions and goals. For some individuals, fasting may not be suitable or may require modifications. It is recommended to consult with a healthcare professional before starting any fasting regimen, especially for pregnant or breastfeeding women, individuals with medical conditions, or those with a history of eating disorders. Additionally, the success of fasting lies in maintaining a balanced and nutritious diet during non-fasting periods to ensure the body receives essential nutrients and sustains overall health.

Debunking Fasting Myths and Misconceptions

Fasting has gained popularity in recent years, and with its rise, various myths and misconceptions have emerged. It is essential to separate fact from fiction to ensure that individuals make informed decisions about fasting and its potential impact on health. Let's debunk some of the common myths surrounding fasting:

Myth 1: Fasting Is Starvation

Fact: Fasting is a voluntary and controlled practice of abstaining from food and, in some cases, beverages for a specific period. It is not the same as starvation, which is an involuntary lack of food and can lead to severe malnutrition and health risks. Fasting is a structured approach that, when done correctly and with proper guidance, can have potential health benefits.

Myth 2: Fasting Slows Down Metabolism

Fact: Short-term fasting does not significantly slow down the metabolism. Fasting can trigger a metabolic switch, leading the body to burn stored fats for energy, a state known as ketosis. This can enhance fat burning and may have positive effects on metabolic health. However, extended fasting without proper nutrition may lead to a temporary reduction in metabolic rate.

Myth 3: Fasting Causes Muscle Loss

Fact: When done appropriately, fasting does not cause significant muscle loss. Short-term fasting can increase human growth hormone (HGH) levels, which supports muscle preservation and repair. It is essential to combine fasting with adequate protein intake and strength training to maintain muscle mass.

Myth 4: Fasting Is Not Safe

Fact: Fasting can be safe for many people when done correctly and under appropriate conditions. However, it may not be suitable for everyone, especially pregnant or breastfeeding women, individuals with certain medical conditions, or those with a history of eating disorders. Consulting a healthcare professional before starting any fasting regimen is essential.

Myth 5: Fasting Leads to Nutrient Deficiencies

Fact: While fasting restricts food intake for a specific period, it does not automatically lead to nutrient deficiencies. A well-planned fasting approach can still provide essential nutrients when balanced with nutrient-rich meals during non-fasting periods. Adequate hydration and a balanced diet are crucial components of a safe and effective fasting plan.

Myth 6: Fasting Is a Quick Fix for Weight Loss

Fact: Fasting can lead to initial weight loss due to reduced calorie intake, but it is not a quick fix. Sustainable weight loss requires a long-term commitment to a balanced diet and a healthy lifestyle that includes regular physical activity.

Myth 7: Fasting Causes Binge Eating

Fact: If fasting is not approached mindfully, it may lead to overeating during non-fasting periods. However, mindful eating practices and incorporating a balanced diet can help prevent binge eating tendencies.

Myth 8: Fasting Is Only for Weight Loss

Fact: While weight loss is one of the potential benefits of fasting, it is not the only reason people practice fasting. Fasting is also used for various health purposes, such as promoting metabolic health, improving insulin sensitivity, and supporting cellular repair through autophagy.

Debunking these myths helps individuals make informed decisions about whether fasting aligns with their health goals and individual circumstances. Like any dietary or lifestyle change, fasting should be approached thoughtfully and with consideration of individual health needs. Consulting a healthcare professional can provide personalized guidance and ensure a safe and effective fasting experience.

Part II

The Science Behind Female Fasting

The Physiology of Women and Fasting

The physiological aspects of women are of significant importance in the context of fasting. The physiological characteristics of women's bodies differ from those of men, primarily as a result of their distinct reproductive system and hormonal variations. These variations have an impact on women's potential responses to fasting and the recommended approach they should adopt towards fasting practices. It is crucial to have a comprehensive understanding of the physiological aspects related to women and fasting in order to develop fasting protocols that effectively support women's overall health and well-being.

1. Menstrual Cycle: One of the fundamental physiological differences between men and women is the menstrual cycle. Throughout the menstrual cycle, hormone levels fluctuate, including estrogen, progesterone, and luteinizing hormone (LH). These hormonal changes can influence energy levels, appetite, and metabolism. Therefore, women may experience fasting differently at different phases of their menstrual cycle.

2. Hormonal Changes: Fasting can affect hormone levels in women, particularly when fasting is extended or practiced inconsistently. Irregular fasting or prolonged fasting may disrupt the menstrual cycle and affect hormonal balance. This highlights the importance of adopting a mindful approach to fasting that considers individual needs and hormonal fluctuations.

3. Impact on Reproductive Health: Women who are trying to conceive, pregnant, or breastfeeding should approach fasting with caution. Caloric restriction and significant changes in eating patterns during fasting can impact reproductive health and the development of a healthy pregnancy. Pregnant and breastfeeding women should prioritize adequate nutrition for themselves and their growing baby.

4. Nutrient Needs: Women generally have different nutrient needs compared to men, especially during specific life stages like pregnancy, breastfeeding, and menopause. Fasting should not compromise essential nutrient intake and should be balanced with nourishing meals during non-fasting periods.

5. Metabolic Differences: Research suggests that women's metabolic responses to fasting may differ from men's. For example, some studies indicate that women's bodies may be more resistant to the effects of fasting on certain metabolic pathways. As a result, women may need to tailor their fasting approach to suit their metabolic responses.

6. Impact on Energy Levels and Mood: Fasting can influence energy levels and mood in both men and women. However, due to women's hormonal fluctuations and potential variations in metabolic responses, fasting may affect energy levels and mood differently in women. Some women may find that fasting supports mental clarity and energy, while others may experience fluctuations in energy and mood during fasting.

7. Bone Health: Women are at a higher risk of osteoporosis compared to men. Prolonged or extreme fasting without sufficient nutrient intake may negatively impact bone health. Adequate calcium, vitamin D, and other essential

nutrients are crucial for maintaining strong and healthy bones in women.

It is crucial to take into account the distinct physiology of women when developing fasting protocols that are in line with their specific health needs and objectives. It is advisable for women to seek guidance from a healthcare professional, especially if they have specific health issues or are contemplating their first experience with fasting. By gaining a comprehensive understanding of how fasting interacts with the physiology of women, individuals can adopt fasting practices that contribute to their overall health and well-being, while also acknowledging and accommodating the unique requirements of their bodies.

Hormones and Fasting

Hormones and fasting share a delicate and intricate relationship, especially in the context of the female body. Hormones are powerful chemical messengers that regulate various physiological processes, including metabolism, hunger, satiety, mood, and reproductive functions. When women engage in fasting, hormonal fluctuations can be influenced, leading to both positive and potentially challenging effects on their overall well-being.

1. Insulin: Fasting can have a significant impact on insulin levels. Insulin is a hormone that helps regulate blood sugar levels by facilitating the uptake of glucose into cells for energy or storage. During fasting, when food intake is reduced or eliminated, insulin levels decrease, leading to lower blood sugar levels and promoting fat burning. Improved insulin sensitivity can be a positive outcome of fasting, helping to prevent insulin resistance and type 2 diabetes.

2. Ghrelin: Ghrelin is often referred to as the "hunger hormone" as it stimulates appetite and increases food intake. During fasting, ghrelin levels tend to rise, leading to increased feelings of hunger. This hormonal response can make fasting challenging, particularly during the initial stages when the body is adjusting to a new eating pattern.

3. Leptin: Leptin is the "satiety hormone," responsible for signaling feelings of fullness and satiety. During fasting, leptin levels may decrease, which can potentially impact appetite regulation. Reduced leptin levels can lead to increased feelings of hunger and a potential risk of overeating during non-fasting periods.

4. Human Growth Hormone (HGH): Fasting triggers an increase in HGH levels, which plays a critical role in metabolism, fat burning, muscle preservation, and overall cellular repair. The elevation of HGH during fasting can be beneficial for women's health and well-being.

5. Cortisol: Cortisol is the primary stress hormone, and its levels can be influenced by fasting. Short-term fasting may lead to moderate increases in cortisol, which is a natural stress response. However, prolonged or extreme fasting may result in persistently elevated cortisol levels, which can have negative effects on the body, including impaired immune function and increased stress.

6. Reproductive Hormones: Fasting, especially when combined with caloric restriction or rapid weight loss, can impact reproductive hormones. For women, disruptions in hormonal balance may affect menstrual cycles, fertility, and reproductive health. Women who are trying to conceive or are experiencing irregular menstrual cycles should approach fasting with caution and seek guidance from a healthcare professional.

Balancing the delicate interplay between hormones and fasting is critical for women's health and well-being. Mindful and responsible fasting practices that prioritize proper nutrition, adequate hydration, and appropriate fasting durations can help maintain hormonal balance and support overall health. Women should consider individual factors, such as age, reproductive status, and health conditions when deciding on the most suitable fasting approach. Consulting with a healthcare provider can provide personalized guidance and ensure that fasting aligns with individual health needs while promoting a harmonious hormonal balance.

How Fasting Impacts Female Metabolism

Fasting can have various impacts on female metabolism, influencing how the body processes and utilizes energy. Understanding these effects is essential for women considering fasting as a part of their health and wellness routine. Here are some ways fasting impacts female metabolism:

1. Ketosis and Fat Burning: During fasting, when the body is deprived of its primary energy source (carbohydrates), it enters a state called ketosis. In ketosis, the body starts breaking down stored fats into ketones, which serve as an alternative source of energy. This process promotes fat burning, making stored fat more accessible for energy expenditure.

2. Metabolic Switch: Fasting triggers a metabolic switch from using glucose as the primary energy source to using fats. This transition can lead to increased fat oxidation and reduced reliance on carbohydrates for energy.

3. Resting Metabolic Rate: Short-term fasting may have minimal impact on resting metabolic rate (RMR), the number of calories burned at rest. However, prolonged or

extreme fasting without adequate nutrition can potentially lead to a reduction in RMR, as the body tries to conserve energy during prolonged periods of calorie restriction.

4. Insulin Sensitivity: Fasting can improve insulin sensitivity, helping the body utilize insulin more efficiently to regulate blood sugar levels. Enhanced insulin sensitivity is beneficial for overall metabolic health and may reduce the risk of insulin resistance and type 2 diabetes.

5. Hormonal Influence: As previously mentioned, fasting can influence hormone levels in women, such as insulin, ghrelin, leptin, and human growth hormone (HGH). These hormonal changes can impact metabolism and appetite regulation.

6. Caloric Intake: Fasting inherently reduces caloric intake, which can lead to a caloric deficit and, subsequently, weight loss. However, women must ensure they consume enough nutrients during non-fasting periods to support their metabolic needs and overall health.

7. Lean Body Mass: Proper fasting, combined with appropriate nutrition and exercise, can help preserve lean body mass. However, extreme fasting or inadequate protein intake may lead to muscle loss, which can negatively impact metabolism over time.

8. Gut Health: Fasting may have positive effects on gut health by promoting a healthier gut microbiota, which plays a role in overall metabolism and digestive function.

9. Hormonal and Metabolic Adaptations: Women may experience unique hormonal and metabolic responses to fasting, particularly due to hormonal fluctuations related to the menstrual cycle. This emphasizes the importance of

adopting a personalized approach to fasting that considers individual needs and responses.

It is essential to approach fasting with mindfulness and prioritize balanced nutrition to support metabolism and overall health. For women, understanding the potential impacts of fasting on their unique physiology and consulting with a healthcare professional can help tailor a fasting regimen that aligns with their health goals and individual needs. Sustainable and responsible fasting practices, when done mindfully, can have positive effects on female metabolism, supporting overall well-being and promoting a healthier lifestyle.

Part III

Preparing for a Successful Fast

Setting Your Intention

Establishing a clear intention and defining specific goals are essential steps for achieving success in fasting. The act of setting intentions can greatly contribute to establishing a sense of focus and motivation, thereby transforming fasting into a purposeful and meaningful endeavor. When establishing your intention for fasting, it is advisable to take the following steps into consideration:

1. Reflect on Your Why: Begin by reflecting on your reasons for incorporating fasting into your lifestyle. Is it for weight loss, improved energy levels, hormonal balance, or other health benefits? Understanding your underlying motivations will provide a strong foundation for your intention.

2. Define Specific Goals: Set clear and realistic goals for your fasting journey. Make your goals specific, measurable, achievable, relevant, and time-bound (SMART). For example, a specific goal could be to lose a certain amount of weight, improve insulin sensitivity, or experience increased mental clarity.

3. Prioritize Health and Well-being: Ensure that your intention emphasizes the importance of health and well-being rather than focusing solely on short-term outcomes like rapid weight loss. Prioritizing overall well-being will help maintain a sustainable and balanced approach to fasting.

4. Consider Your Individual Needs: Recognize that fasting is not a one-size-fits-all approach. Consider your age, health status, lifestyle, and any specific health conditions when setting your intention. Personalizing your fasting plan will enhance its effectiveness and safety.

5. Create a Plan: Once you have defined your intention and goals, create a detailed fasting plan. Decide on the fasting method that aligns with your objectives, such as intermittent fasting, time-restricted eating, or alternate-day fasting. Determine the fasting schedule, duration, and eating window that suits your lifestyle and preferences.

6. Seek Professional Guidance: If you have specific health concerns or are new to fasting, consider consulting a healthcare professional or a registered dietitian. They can offer personalized advice, address any health considerations, and help design a fasting plan that supports your well-being.

7. Monitor and Adjust: Regularly monitor your progress toward your fasting goals. Keep a journal to record how you feel, any changes you observe, and your overall experience with fasting. Based on your observations, be open to adjusting your fasting plan as needed to optimize your results.

8. Cultivate Mindfulness: Practice mindfulness during fasting to stay connected with your body and emotions. Listen to your body's hunger and satiety cues, and respect its signals. Mindful eating during non-fasting periods is equally essential to nourish your body optimally.

9. Practice Self-Compassion: Fasting can present challenges, especially during the adjustment phase. Practice self-compassion and avoid being too hard on yourself if things

don't go perfectly. Be patient and recognize that fasting is a journey, and it's okay to make adjustments along the way.

10. Celebrate Achievements: Acknowledge and celebrate your fasting achievements, no matter how small they may seem. Celebrating progress can reinforce positive habits and keep you motivated to continue on your fasting journey.

Setting a clear intention and goal setting for fasting success empowers you to approach fasting with purpose and mindfulness. With a well-defined plan and a focus on your overall well-being, you can make fasting a positive and transformative experience that aligns with your health goals and enhances your quality of life.

Creating a Safe and Effective Fasting Plan

Creating a safe and effective fasting plan requires careful consideration of individual health factors, lifestyle, and goals. Follow these steps to develop a fasting plan that supports your well-being and maximizes the potential benefits:

1. Assess Your Health: Before starting any fasting regimen, assess your health status and consider any medical conditions you may have. Consult with a healthcare professional to ensure fasting is safe and appropriate for you. This is especially important if you have diabetes, thyroid disorders, hormonal imbalances, or any other health concerns.

2. Choose the Right Fasting Method: Select a fasting method that aligns with your goals and lifestyle. Common approaches include intermittent fasting (e.g., 16/8, 5:2), time-restricted eating, or alternate-day fasting. Start with a less restrictive method if you are new to fasting.

3. Gradual Transition: If you are new to fasting, consider easing into it with a gradual transition. Begin by extending the time between your last meal of the day and your first meal the next day. Slowly increase the fasting duration as your body adapts.

4. Stay Hydrated: Drink plenty of water during fasting periods to stay hydrated. Avoid beverages with added sugars or calories, as they can break the fast.

5. Choose Nutrient-Dense Foods: Prioritize nutrient-dense foods during non-fasting periods to support your body's needs. Include a variety of vegetables, fruits, whole grains, lean proteins, and healthy fats in your meals.

6. Pay Attention to Portion Sizes: Avoid overeating during non-fasting periods, as it can counteract the benefits of fasting. Be mindful of portion sizes and listen to your body's hunger and satiety cues.

7. Monitor Your Energy Levels: Pay attention to how your body responds to fasting. If you feel fatigued or experience dizziness, consider modifying your fasting plan or consulting a healthcare professional.

8. Customize Your Schedule: Tailor your fasting schedule to fit your daily routine and lifestyle. It's essential to find a plan that is sustainable and convenient for you.

9. Be Flexible: Allow room for flexibility in your fasting plan. Life events and special occasions may require adjustments to your fasting schedule. Being flexible helps you maintain a balanced approach to fasting.

10. Listen to Your Body: Above all, listen to your body and be responsive to its needs. If fasting feels too challenging or

uncomfortable, consider modifying your approach or trying a different fasting method.

11. Avoid Extreme Fasting: Extreme fasting, such as prolonged water fasting or severely restricted calorie intake, can be dangerous and may lead to nutrient deficiencies and other health risks. Avoid extreme fasting without medical supervision.

12. Regular Check-Ins: Regularly assess your progress and how you feel during fasting. Keep a journal to track any changes in your energy, mood, and overall well-being.

By creating a safe and effective fasting plan tailored to your needs, you can optimize the potential benefits of fasting while promoting your overall health and well-being. Remember that fasting may not be suitable for everyone, and individual experiences can vary. If you have any concerns or questions about fasting, seek guidance from a healthcare professional before starting your fasting journey.

Overcoming Common Challenges in Female Fasting

Fasting can present unique challenges for women due to their hormonal fluctuations, reproductive health, and metabolic differences. Overcoming these challenges is essential to ensure a safe and positive fasting experience. Here are some strategies to address common challenges in female fasting:

1. Managing Hunger: Women may experience increased feelings of hunger during fasting, especially during certain phases of their menstrual cycle. To manage hunger, consider starting with shorter fasting periods and gradually extending them as your body adapts. Stay hydrated with water or herbal teas to help reduce hunger cues.

2. Balancing Hormones: Hormonal changes during fasting can impact mood and energy levels. Prioritize self-care practices, such as meditation, yoga, and relaxation techniques, to support emotional well-being during fasting. Adequate sleep is also crucial for hormone balance.

3. Avoiding Extreme Fasting: Extreme fasting or prolonged fasting without adequate nutrition can be detrimental to women's health. Avoid drastic calorie restriction or extended water fasting, especially if you have specific health concerns.

4. Mindful Eating: Practice mindful eating during non-fasting periods to ensure you consume balanced and nutrient-dense meals. Avoid binge-eating after fasting, as it can lead to discomfort and disrupt the metabolic balance.

5. Nourishing Your Body: Focus on nutrient-dense foods that provide essential vitamins and minerals during non-fasting periods. Prioritize whole grains, lean proteins, fruits, vegetables, and healthy fats to support overall health.

6. Adjusting Fasting Schedule: Be flexible with your fasting schedule to accommodate hormonal fluctuations or life events. Consider adapting your fasting plan based on how you feel during different phases of your menstrual cycle.

7. Stay Hydrated: Hydration is essential during fasting to support metabolic processes and overall well-being. Drink plenty of water and herbal teas during fasting periods.

8. Seeking Support: Join a community or find a fasting buddy to share experiences, tips, and motivation. Connecting with others can provide support and encouragement during your fasting journey.

9. Avoid Fasting During Pregnancy: Fasting during pregnancy is not recommended, as it may negatively impact maternal and fetal health. Focus on a balanced and nutritious diet during pregnancy to support both you and your baby.

10. Consulting a Healthcare Professional: If you have specific health concerns, are pregnant, breastfeeding, or have a history of eating disorders, consult with a healthcare professional before starting any fasting regimen.

11. Being Patient: Be patient with yourself and your body during fasting. Allow time for adaptation and listen to your body's needs. If fasting feels overwhelming, consider adjusting your approach or trying a different fasting method.

12. Focus on Overall Well-being: Remember that fasting is just one aspect of a healthy lifestyle. Prioritize overall well-being by incorporating regular physical activity, adequate sleep, and stress management practices into your routine.

By being mindful of these challenges and adopting a balanced approach to fasting, women can overcome obstacles and embrace fasting as a tool to support their health and well-being. Remember that fasting is a personal journey, and it's essential to honor your body's unique needs and responses throughout the process.

Part IV

Fasting for Weight Loss and Fat Burning

Fasting for Weight Loss

Fasting can be an effective strategy for weight loss when done safely and mindfully. Here are some best practices and strategies for using fasting as a tool for weight loss:

1. Choose a Fasting Method: Select a fasting method that aligns with your lifestyle and preferences. Intermittent fasting (e.g., 16/8, 5:2), time-restricted eating, or alternate-day fasting are popular options for weight loss.

2. Start Gradually: If you are new to fasting, start with a gradual approach. Begin with shorter fasting periods and gradually increase the duration as your body adapts. This can help minimize potential side effects and make fasting more sustainable.

3. Focus on Nutrient-Dense Foods: During non-fasting periods, prioritize nutrient-dense foods that provide essential vitamins and minerals. Include a variety of vegetables, fruits, whole grains, lean proteins, and healthy fats in your meals.

4. Be Mindful of Portions: Pay attention to portion sizes during non-fasting periods to avoid overeating and negate the benefits of fasting. Listen to your body's hunger and satiety cues.

5. Stay Hydrated: Drink plenty of water and herbal teas during fasting periods to stay hydrated. Avoid caloric

beverages like sugary sodas or fruit juices that can break the fast.

6. Be Mindful of Your Body's Response: Pay attention to how your body responds to fasting. If you experience significant discomfort, fatigue, or dizziness, consider modifying your fasting plan or consulting a healthcare professional.

7. Monitor Your Progress: Keep a journal to track your weight loss progress and how you feel during fasting. This can help you assess the effectiveness of your fasting plan and make any necessary adjustments.

8. Include Physical Activity: Combine fasting with regular physical activity to enhance weight loss and overall health. Choose activities you enjoy, such as walking, jogging, dancing, or yoga.

9. Avoid Overcompensation: After fasting, avoid overcompensating by binge-eating or consuming excessive calories. Stick to balanced and portion-controlled meals during non-fasting periods.

10. Stay Consistent: Consistency is key to weight loss success. Stick to your fasting schedule and maintain a healthy diet to achieve sustainable results.

11. Avoid Extreme Fasting: Extreme fasting or prolonged water fasting is not recommended for weight loss, as it can lead to nutrient deficiencies and metabolic imbalances. Choose a moderate fasting approach that is safe and sustainable.

12. Seek Support: Joining a fasting community or finding a fasting buddy can provide support, motivation, and accountability during your weight loss journey.

Remember that weight loss is a gradual process, and individual results may vary. Be patient with yourself, and avoid comparing your progress to others. Fasting for weight loss should be done in conjunction with a balanced diet and lifestyle to achieve sustainable and long-term results. If you have any health concerns or medical conditions, consult with a healthcare professional before starting any fasting regimen.

The Role of Autophagy in Fat Burning

Autophagy plays a significant role in fat-burning and overall metabolic health. Autophagy is a cellular process that involves the breakdown and recycling of damaged or dysfunctional cellular components, including proteins, organelles, and other cellular debris. This process is crucial for maintaining cellular health and homeostasis. Autophagy has been linked to various health benefits, including its impact on fat metabolism.

1. Fat Utilization: During autophagy, the body breaks down and recycles cellular components, including lipids (fats). This process increases the availability of fatty acids for energy production. As a result, autophagy promotes the utilization of stored fats for energy, contributing to fat burning.

2. Ketogenesis: Autophagy can trigger ketogenesis, the process by which the liver produces ketone bodies from fats. Ketones serve as an alternative energy source when carbohydrates are scarce, such as during fasting or a low-carb diet. Ketones are particularly beneficial for brain function, as they can cross the blood-brain barrier and provide energy to the brain during periods of fasting or carbohydrate restriction.

3. Insulin Sensitivity: Autophagy has been shown to improve insulin sensitivity, which is essential for healthy glucose metabolism and weight management. Improved insulin sensitivity helps the body use insulin more effectively, reducing the risk of insulin resistance and type 2 diabetes.

4. Weight Loss: Autophagy's role in promoting fat burning and improving metabolic health can contribute to weight loss. When the body efficiently utilizes stored fats for energy, it can lead to a reduction in body fat over time, particularly when combined with a balanced diet and regular physical activity.

5. Cellular Repair: By eliminating damaged cellular components, autophagy supports cellular repair and renewal. This process is essential for overall cellular health and can help optimize cellular function and metabolism.

6. Longevity: Autophagy has been associated with longevity and aging. By clearing out damaged cellular components, autophagy may contribute to cellular longevity and potentially slow down the aging process.

Autophagy is primarily triggered during periods of cellular stress, such as fasting, caloric restriction, or exercise. Fasting, in particular, is a potent stimulator of autophagy. During fasting, the body depletes its carbohydrate stores, leading to a decrease in insulin levels and an increase in glucagon levels. Glucagon is a hormone that promotes autophagy and fat breakdown.

Combining Fasting with Exercise for Optimal Results

Combining fasting with exercise can be a powerful strategy for achieving optimal results in terms of weight loss, metabolic health, and overall well-being. When done correctly and mindfully, this combination can complement each other and enhance the benefits of both fasting and exercise. Here are some tips for combining fasting with exercise for optimal results:

1. Choose the Right Exercise: Select exercises that suit your fitness level and preferences. Incorporate a mix of cardiovascular exercises (e.g., walking, jogging, cycling) and strength training (e.g., weightlifting, bodyweight exercises) to improve overall fitness and support fat burning.

2. Time Your Workouts: Schedule your exercise sessions during non-fasting periods to ensure you have enough energy and stamina to perform your workouts effectively. If you practice time-restricted eating, plan your workouts during your eating window.

3. Moderate Intensity: During fasting periods, opt for moderate-intensity exercises to avoid excessive strain on the body. High-intensity workouts may be more challenging to sustain during fasting and can lead to fatigue.

4. Stay Hydrated: Hydration is essential, especially when combining fasting with exercise. Drink plenty of water before, during, and after your workouts to stay hydrated and support your performance.

5. Pre-Workout Nutrition: If your fasting window aligns with your exercise session, consider consuming a small, balanced snack before your workout. This can provide the necessary fuel without breaking your fast. Examples include a piece of fruit, a handful of nuts, or a protein shake.

6. Post-Workout Nutrition: After your workout, prioritize nutrient-dense foods to support recovery and muscle repair. Include protein-rich foods, healthy carbohydrates, and a moderate amount of healthy fats in your post-workout meal.

7. Listen to Your Body: Pay attention to how your body responds to exercise during fasting. If you feel excessively fatigued or lightheaded, consider modifying the intensity or timing of your workouts.

8. Consider Fasted Workouts: Some individuals prefer fasted workouts, where they exercise during the fasting period. Fasted workouts may enhance fat burning since the body relies more on stored fats for energy. Experiment with fasted workouts to see how your body responds.

9. Plan Rest Days: Incorporate rest days into your exercise routine to allow your body to recover and prevent overtraining, especially when fasting.

10. Be Mindful of Macronutrients: When combining fasting with exercise, ensure you are getting adequate protein to support muscle recovery and growth. Protein intake is essential, especially if you are engaging in strength training.

11. Avoid Overcompensation: Be cautious of overeating or rewarding yourself with unhealthy foods after exercise. Be mindful of your nutritional choices during non-fasting periods to support your weight loss and health goals.

12. Monitor Progress: Keep track of your progress regarding weight loss, fitness gains, and overall well-being to assess the effectiveness of combining fasting with exercise.

Part V

Fasting for Energy and Performance

Harnessing the Power of Fasting for Increased Energy Levels

Fasting can be a powerful tool for increasing energy levels when done correctly and mindfully. By promoting fat burning, improving insulin sensitivity, and supporting cellular repair, fasting can lead to enhanced energy and vitality. Here are some strategies to harness the power of fasting for increased energy levels:

1. Start Gradually: If you are new to fasting, begin with a gradual approach. Start with shorter fasting periods and gradually increase the duration as your body adapts. Sudden and extreme changes in eating patterns can lead to fatigue and discomfort.

2. Stay Hydrated: Proper hydration is essential during fasting to maintain energy levels. Drink plenty of water and herbal teas throughout the day to stay hydrated. Dehydration can contribute to feelings of tiredness.

3. Choose Nutrient-Dense Foods: During non-fasting periods, focus on consuming nutrient-dense foods that provide essential vitamins and minerals. Include a variety of vegetables, fruits, whole grains, lean proteins, and healthy fats in your meals to support energy production.

4. Time Your Fasting: Consider timing your fasting periods to align with your natural energy peaks and dips. Some individuals find that fasting in the morning or early afternoon works best for them, while others prefer fasting in the evening.

5. Listen to Your Body: Pay attention to how your body responds to fasting. If you feel excessively fatigued or lightheaded, consider modifying your fasting plan or seeking guidance from a healthcare professional.

6. Optimize Sleep: Ensure you are getting enough quality sleep during fasting periods. Sleep is crucial for energy restoration and overall well-being. Establish a consistent sleep schedule and create a relaxing bedtime routine.

7. Include Light Exercise: Engage in light to moderate exercise during fasting periods, such as walking or gentle yoga. Exercise can boost energy levels and promote mental clarity.

8. Mindful Eating: Practice mindful eating during non-fasting periods. Eat slowly, savor your meals, and pay attention to hunger and satiety cues. Overeating during non-fasting periods can lead to energy fluctuations.

9. Manage Stress: High levels of stress can deplete energy reserves. Practice stress-reducing techniques such as meditation, deep breathing, or spending time in nature to manage stress during fasting.

10. Monitor Your Progress: Keep a journal to track your energy levels and overall experience with fasting. Monitoring your progress can help you identify patterns and make adjustments as needed.

11. Avoid Overcompensation: After fasting, avoid overcompensating by consuming excessive calories or unhealthy foods. Focus on balanced and nourishing meals during non-fasting periods.

12. Consult a Healthcare Professional: If you have specific health concerns or medical conditions, consult with a

healthcare professional before starting any fasting regimen to ensure it aligns with your individual needs.

Remember that the effects of fasting on energy levels may vary among individuals. Some people may experience an increase in energy, while others may require time to adapt. Be patient with yourself and find a fasting approach that works best for you and supports your energy and overall health goals.

Fasting for Physical and Mental Performance

Fasting can have notable effects on both physical and mental performance. When done mindfully and appropriately, fasting can enhance energy metabolism, promote fat utilization, and improve cognitive function.

Physically, fasting triggers the body to rely on stored fat for energy, leading to increased fat burning. This can be beneficial for individuals aiming to improve body composition or enhance athletic performance. Moreover, fasting may boost human growth hormone (HGH) levels, promoting muscle preservation and growth.

On the mental front, fasting has been linked to improved cognitive function and mental clarity. During fasting, the brain utilizes ketones as an alternative energy source, which may lead to enhanced focus and concentration. Additionally, fasting can activate autophagy, a cellular process that supports brain health and neuronal repair.

However, it is important to note that the effects of fasting on performance can vary among individuals. Proper hydration and balanced nutrition during non-fasting periods are essential to support physical and mental well-being. Furthermore, individuals with specific health concerns or medical conditions should consult with healthcare professionals before implementing fasting for performance enhancement. By adopting a mindful and individualized approach, individuals may harness the potential benefits of fasting to optimize physical and mental performance.

Fasting for Improved Athletic Performance

Fasting has gained popularity as a potential strategy to enhance athletic performance, especially among endurance athletes. When applied correctly, fasting can offer several benefits that may positively impact athletic performance. Here are some ways fasting may improve athletic performance:

1. Enhanced Fat Utilization: Fasting can promote the body's ability to use stored fats as a primary source of energy during exercise. This is particularly advantageous for endurance athletes who often rely on fat oxidation during prolonged activities, such as long-distance running or cycling.

2. Improved Insulin Sensitivity: Fasting can lead to improved insulin sensitivity, which helps the body utilize carbohydrates more efficiently during exercise. This may result in better glycogen storage and utilization, crucial for high-intensity efforts and prolonged activities.

3. Increased Human Growth Hormone (HGH) Levels: Fasting triggers an increase in HGH levels, which can support muscle preservation and growth. This may be beneficial for athletes looking to optimize their muscle mass-to-fat ratio.

4. Autophagy and Cellular Repair: Fasting promotes autophagy, a cellular process that facilitates the removal of

damaged cellular components. This may lead to better cellular health, recovery, and overall athletic performance.

5. Mental Clarity and Focus: Some athletes report improved mental clarity and focus during fasting, which can be advantageous for maintaining concentration and determination during training and competition.

6. Training Adaptations: Periodic fasting, when combined with proper nutrition, can create a hormetic effect, stimulating the body's adaptive responses to stress. This may lead to improved training adaptations and performance gains.

7. Weight Management: Fasting can support weight management and body composition, which may be relevant for athletes in weight-sensitive sports.

However, it is essential to approach fasting for improved athletic performance with caution and individualization. Athletes have varying energy requirements and nutritional needs, and fasting may not be suitable for everyone. Factors such as training volume, intensity, sport type, and individual health status should be considered when incorporating fasting into an athlete's regimen.

Additionally, the timing and duration of fasting should be carefully planned to ensure athletes have sufficient energy for training and recovery. Fasting should not compromise an athlete's overall nutrition and hydration status, and athletes must prioritize proper nutrient intake during non-fasting periods.

Part VI

Fasting for Hormonal Balance

The Impact of Fasting on Hormonal Health

Fasting can have a significant impact on hormonal health, influencing the delicate balance of various hormones in the body. Hormones are powerful chemical messengers that regulate numerous physiological processes, and their fluctuations during fasting play a crucial role in the overall effects of fasting on health and well-being. Here are some of the key ways fasting can impact hormonal health:

1. Insulin: Fasting can lead to reduced insulin levels in the blood, as the body adapts to lower glucose availability. Improved insulin sensitivity is often observed during fasting, which can be beneficial for individuals at risk of insulin resistance and type 2 diabetes.

2. Ghrelin: Ghrelin, also known as the "hunger hormone," increases during fasting. The rise in ghrelin levels signals the body's hunger response, which may lead to increased appetite and food intake during non-fasting periods.

3. Leptin: Leptin, the "satiety hormone," may decrease during fasting. This reduction can impact hunger regulation, potentially leading to increased feelings of hunger and the risk of overeating during refeeding.

4. Human Growth Hormone (HGH): Fasting triggers an increase in HGH levels, promoting cellular repair, fat metabolism, and muscle preservation. The elevation of

HGH during fasting can have positive effects on body composition and overall health.

5. Cortisol: Short-term fasting may lead to moderate increases in cortisol, the stress hormone. This is a natural adaptive response to fasting. However, prolonged or extreme fasting may result in persistently elevated cortisol levels, which can have negative effects on immune function and overall well-being.

6. Thyroid Hormones: Some studies suggest that prolonged or extreme fasting can lead to reduced levels of thyroid hormones, potentially impacting metabolism. However, this effect is usually observed in cases of severe caloric restriction and prolonged fasting.

7. Reproductive Hormones: Fasting can influence reproductive hormones, especially in women. Extreme or inadequate fasting may lead to disruptions in menstrual cycles and reproductive health. Women trying to conceive or experiencing irregular menstrual cycles should approach fasting with caution and seek guidance from a healthcare professional.

8. Adiponectin: Fasting can increase adiponectin levels, a hormone involved in regulating glucose and lipid metabolism. Higher adiponectin levels are associated with improved insulin sensitivity and reduced inflammation.

It's important to note that the hormonal response to fasting can vary among individuals, and the effects of fasting on hormone levels may depend on factors such as fasting duration, frequency, and individual health status.

To promote hormonal health while fasting, it's essential to adopt a mindful and balanced approach to fasting. Gradual fasting protocols, proper hydration, and balanced nutrient intake during non-fasting periods are crucial for supporting hormonal balance and overall well-being. As with any significant dietary or lifestyle changes, individuals with specific health concerns or medical conditions should consult with a healthcare professional before starting a fasting regimen.

Fasting to Regulate Menstrual Cycles and PMS Symptoms

Fasting can have both positive and negative effects on menstrual cycles and premenstrual syndrome (PMS) symptoms in women. While some women may find that fasting helps regulate their menstrual cycles and reduces PMS symptoms, others may experience disruptions or worsening of symptoms. Here's how fasting can impact menstrual health:

1. Hormonal Balance: Fasting can influence hormone levels, including estrogen, progesterone, and other reproductive hormones. For some women, fasting may promote hormonal balance and regular menstrual cycles, potentially leading to reduced PMS symptoms.

2. Insulin Sensitivity: Fasting may improve insulin sensitivity, which can be beneficial for women with polycystic ovary syndrome (PCOS) or insulin resistance-related menstrual irregularities.

3. Weight Management: Fasting can support weight management, and maintaining a healthy weight is associated with improved menstrual regularity and reduced PMS symptoms.

4. Autophagy and Cellular Repair: Fasting promotes cellular repair, which may positively impact overall reproductive health.

However, it's essential to approach fasting for menstrual health with caution and individualization:

1. Impact on Reproductive Hormones: Extreme or inadequate fasting can disrupt reproductive hormone levels, leading to irregular menstrual cycles or amenorrhea (absence of periods). Women trying to regulate their cycles or manage PMS symptoms through fasting should adopt a moderate fasting approach and ensure they are meeting their nutritional needs during non-fasting periods.

2. Nutrient Intake: Insufficient nutrient intake during fasting can negatively affect reproductive health. Women should prioritize nutrient-dense foods and proper hydration during non-fasting periods to support their menstrual health.

3. Individual Variability: Women's responses to fasting can vary widely. Some may experience improvements in their menstrual health, while others may experience adverse effects. Pay attention to how your body responds and consider consulting a healthcare professional if you have concerns.

4. Stress and Hormones: Prolonged or chronic fasting-related stress can lead to elevated cortisol levels, which can disrupt reproductive hormones and menstrual cycles.

5. Fasting Length and Frequency: The duration and frequency of fasting can impact menstrual health. Women should experiment with different fasting schedules to find what works best for them.

If you have irregular menstrual cycles, PMS symptoms, or any reproductive health concerns, it's essential to consult with a healthcare professional or a registered dietitian before incorporating fasting into your routine. They can help you develop a personalized approach that supports your reproductive health while taking into account your individual needs and goals. In some cases, fasting may not be suitable, and other lifestyle modifications or treatments may be more appropriate for managing menstrual health and PMS symptoms.

Managing Menopause and Hormonal Changes through Fasting

Managing menopause and hormonal changes through fasting requires careful consideration and a personalized approach. Menopause is a natural biological process that marks the end of a woman's reproductive years and is characterized by hormonal fluctuations, specifically a decline in estrogen and progesterone levels. While fasting may offer some potential benefits during menopause, it is essential to approach it with mindfulness and adaptability. Here are some considerations for managing menopause through fasting:

1. Consult a Healthcare Professional: Before incorporating fasting into your routine during menopause, consult with a healthcare professional, such as a gynecologist or a registered dietitian. They can assess your health status and provide personalized guidance on whether fasting is suitable for you.

2. Balance Hormonal Changes: Menopause can lead to various symptoms, including hot flashes, mood swings, and sleep disturbances. Focus on a balanced approach to fasting and prioritize nutrient-dense foods to support hormonal balance and overall well-being.

3. Adjust Fasting Schedule: Women experiencing menopause may find that fasting affects their energy levels or exacerbates certain symptoms. Be open to adjusting your fasting schedule as needed to suit your body's changing needs.

4. Bone Health: Estrogen plays a crucial role in maintaining bone density, and its decline during menopause can increase the risk of osteoporosis. Ensure adequate calcium and vitamin D intake during non-fasting periods to support bone health.

5. Heart Health: Menopause is associated with an increased risk of cardiovascular issues. While fasting can have benefits for heart health, ensure a well-rounded approach that includes regular physical activity and heart-healthy foods.

6. Monitor Stress Levels: Menopause can be a time of increased stress, and fasting-related stress may exacerbate symptoms. Manage stress through mindfulness practices, relaxation techniques, and stress-reducing activities.

7. Hydration: Stay well-hydrated during fasting and non-fasting periods to support overall health and mitigate potential menopause-related symptoms.

8. Be Gentle with Yourself: Menopause is a natural transition, and every woman's experience is unique. Be patient with yourself and allow room for flexibility in your fasting approach.

9. Address Individual Needs: Some women may find that fasting is not well-tolerated during menopause, while others may experience benefits. Listen to your body's cues and make adjustments accordingly.

10. Focus on Whole Foods: Prioritize whole, unprocessed foods during non-fasting periods to provide your body with essential nutrients and support overall health.

Remember that fasting is just one aspect of a healthy lifestyle, and it may not be the right approach for everyone during menopause. Prioritize self-care, maintain open communication with healthcare professionals, and consider other lifestyle factors such as exercise, sleep, and stress management to support your well-being during this life stage.

Part VII

Integrating Fasting into Your Lifestyle

Building a Sustainable Fasting Routine

Building a sustainable fasting routine involves creating a plan that is safe, effective, and adaptable to your lifestyle and individual needs. To develop a fasting routine that you can maintain in the long term, consider the following steps:

1. Understand Your Goals: Determine your objectives for fasting. Whether it's weight management, improved metabolic health, or other health benefits, clarifying your goals will help shape your fasting approach.

2. Start Gradually: If you are new to fasting, begin with a gentle approach. Consider starting with time-restricted eating, such as a 12-hour fasting window, and gradually increase the fasting duration as you become more comfortable.

3. Choose a Fasting Method: Explore different fasting methods, such as intermittent fasting, alternate-day fasting, or time-restricted eating, and select one that suits your preferences and fits well with your daily routine.

4. Be Mindful of Your Body: Pay attention to how your body responds to fasting. If you experience excessive fatigue, dizziness, or discomfort, consider modifying your fasting schedule or seeking guidance from a healthcare professional.

5. Prioritize Nutrient-Dense Foods: During non-fasting periods, focus on consuming balanced and nutrient-dense

meals that provide essential vitamins and minerals. Avoid excessive indulgence or overeating after fasting periods.

6. Stay Hydrated: Drink plenty of water and herbal teas throughout the day, especially during fasting periods, to stay hydrated and support your body's functions.

7. Plan Fasting Around Your Lifestyle: Choose a fasting schedule that aligns with your daily activities and social commitments. Be flexible and adapt your fasting routine when necessary.

8. Set Realistic Expectations: Understand that the results of fasting can vary among individuals. Set realistic expectations and focus on the overall health benefits of fasting rather than solely on weight loss.

9. Monitor Your Progress: Keep track of your fasting routine, energy levels, and overall well-being. Regularly assess how fasting impacts your goals and make adjustments as needed.

10. Incorporate Physical Activity: Combine fasting with regular physical activity to support your health and well-being. Engage in exercises that you enjoy and that align with your fasting schedule.

11. Practice Mindfulness: Be mindful of your relationship with food and eating habits. Avoid using fasting as a way to compensate for unhealthy eating patterns or as a means of punishment for overeating.

12. Seek Support: Connect with a community of individuals who practice fasting or find a fasting buddy. Support and accountability can be valuable in maintaining a sustainable fasting routine.

Remember that sustainable fasting is about finding a balanced approach that works for you, supports your health goals, and fits seamlessly into your lifestyle. If you have specific health concerns or medical conditions, consult with a healthcare professional or a registered dietitian before starting any fasting regimen. They can provide personalized guidance and recommendations to ensure that your fasting routine is safe and tailored to your needs.

Combining Fasting with Other Dietary Approaches

Combining fasting with other dietary approaches can be a powerful strategy to optimize health and achieve specific goals. Fasting can complement various dietary patterns and enhance their benefits. Here are some popular dietary approaches that can be combined with fasting:

1. Ketogenic Diet and Intermittent Fasting: The ketogenic diet involves consuming a high-fat, low-carbohydrate diet, which promotes the production of ketones for energy. Intermittent fasting can further enhance ketone production and fat burning, making it an effective combination for weight loss, improved metabolic health, and mental clarity.

2. Plant-Based Diet and Time-Restricted Eating: A plant-based diet focuses on whole, plant foods and avoids animal products. Combining it with time-restricted eating (e.g., 16/8) can enhance nutrient absorption and support the body's natural circadian rhythm, potentially improving digestion, energy levels, and overall health.

3. Mediterranean Diet and Alternate-Day Fasting: The Mediterranean diet emphasizes fruits, vegetables, whole grains, healthy fats, and lean proteins. Combining it with alternate-day fasting (e.g., fasting every other day) can

promote weight loss and heart health while enjoying the diverse and delicious Mediterranean cuisine.

4. Paleo Diet and Extended Fasting: The paleo diet emphasizes foods that our ancestors likely ate during the Paleolithic era, such as meats, fish, fruits, vegetables, nuts, and seeds. Combining it with occasional extended fasting (e.g., 24-48 hours) can mimic periods of food scarcity experienced by early humans and promote metabolic flexibility.

5. Whole Foods Diet and Weekly Fasting: A whole foods diet focuses on minimally processed, nutrient-dense foods. Pairing it with a weekly fasting schedule (e.g., 5:2 fasting) can enhance the benefits of whole foods by promoting cellular repair, reducing inflammation, and supporting weight management.

6. Flexitarian Diet and Modified Fasting: The flexitarian diet is a flexible, plant-based approach that occasionally includes meat and animal products. Pairing it with modified fasting (e.g., fasting on specific days of the week) allows for customization while still reaping the benefits of fasting.

7. DASH Diet and Time-Restricted Eating: The Dietary Approach to Stop Hypertension (DASH) diet emphasizes fruits, vegetables, whole grains, and lean proteins to lower blood pressure. Combining it with time-restricted eating can support cardiovascular health and weight management.

When combining fasting with other dietary approaches, it's crucial to prioritize nutrient intake during non-fasting periods to ensure that your body receives essential vitamins, minerals, and macronutrients. Additionally, listen to your body's cues, be mindful of any individual health conditions or concerns, and consider seeking guidance from a healthcare professional or registered dietitian to create a personalized and sustainable plan that meets your specific needs and goals.

Navigating Social Situations and Maintaining Fasting Consistency

Navigating social situations while fasting can present some challenges, but with planning and mindful choices, you can maintain fasting consistency without feeling deprived or isolated. Here are some strategies to help you stay on track during social events:

1. Plan Ahead: Before attending social gatherings, check the event schedule to identify potential fasting-friendly periods. Plan your fasting windows accordingly, so they align with meal times during the event.

2. Communicate with Others: Inform close friends or family members about your fasting routine and why it is essential to you. This can help them understand and respect your choices, reducing any pressure to break your fast.

3. Bring Your Fasting-Friendly Snacks: If you know that there might not be suitable fasting-friendly options available, bring snacks that align with your fasting plan. Nuts, seeds, and low-carb vegetables can be convenient choices.

4. Hydrate: Stay hydrated during social events by drinking water or unsweetened herbal teas. Hydration can help manage hunger and keep you feeling more satisfied during fasting periods.

5. Practice Mindful Eating: If you choose to eat during a social event, practice mindful eating. Focus on enjoying the flavors and textures of your food, and listen to your body's hunger and satiety cues.

6. Opt for Fasting-Friendly Foods: Look for fasting-friendly options on the menu, such as salads with lean protein, vegetable-based dishes, or broths. Avoid sugary beverages and high-calorie snacks that can disrupt your fasting plan.

7. Be Confident in Your Choices: Remember that your fasting routine is a personal choice, and you have the right to make decisions that support your health and well-being. Be confident in explaining your choices to others if necessary.

8. Avoid Peer Pressure: Social situations can involve peer pressure to eat or drink. Politely decline if you are fasting, and assertively explain your decision without feeling guilty or embarrassed.

9. Focus on Social Interaction: Engage in conversations and activities during the event to take your mind off food. Socializing can distract you from any temptations to break your fast prematurely.

10. Prepare for Fasting Breaks: If you plan to break your fast during the social event, decide in advance when and what you will eat. Make mindful choices and avoid overindulging.

11. Forgive Yourself for Slip-Ups: If you unintentionally break your fast during a social event, don't be too hard on yourself. Acknowledge the slip-up and resume your fasting routine without feeling discouraged.

Remember that maintaining fasting consistency during social events is about finding a balance that works for you and aligns with your health goals. Be flexible, adapt to different situations, and prioritize your well-being while still enjoying social gatherings. Over time, you'll develop a better understanding of how to navigate social situations while sticking to your fasting routine.

Conclusion

Embracing the Journey of Fasting

Embracing the journey of fasting is an empowering and transformative experience that goes beyond just a dietary practice. Fasting offers an opportunity for self-discovery, self-discipline, and improved overall well-being. Here are some ways to embrace the journey of fasting:

1. Mindful Awareness: Approach fasting with mindful awareness of your body's needs and responses. Pay attention to how fasting impacts your energy levels, mood, and overall health. Embrace the changes and be open to learning from the experience.

2. Set Intentions: Establish clear intentions for your fasting journey. Whether it's for weight management, improved metabolic health, or mental clarity, having well-defined goals can give purpose and direction to your fasting practice.

3. Focus on Health, Not Perfection: Embrace fasting as a tool for better health and well-being, rather than striving for perfection or extreme results. Celebrate the progress you make along the way, no matter how small.

4. Learn from Challenges: Fasting may present challenges, both physically and mentally. Embrace these challenges as opportunities for growth and self-improvement. Learn from setbacks and use them to refine your fasting approach.

5. Practice Self-Compassion: Be kind to yourself during the fasting journey. Understand that fasting is a personal process, and it's okay to have ups and downs. Show

yourself compassion and treat yourself with the same understanding you would offer to a friend.

6. Embrace Flexibility: Fasting does not have to be rigid. Embrace flexibility in your fasting routine to accommodate social events, travel, or unexpected situations. The key is to find a sustainable approach that fits your lifestyle.

7. Celebrate Non-Food Benefits: Embrace the non-food benefits of fasting. Improved mental clarity, increased mindfulness, and a sense of empowerment are just a few of the positive outcomes you may experience.

8. Cultivate Gratitude: Practice gratitude for the ability to choose fasting as a part of your wellness journey. Appreciate the abundance of food and nourishment available to you and approach fasting from a place of gratitude.

9. Connect with Others: Engage with a community of like-minded individuals who also practice fasting. Share experiences, challenges, and successes to gain support and encouragement along the way.

10. Embrace the Process: Embrace fasting as a journey rather than a destination. The path to improved health and well-being is ongoing and ever-evolving. Embrace the process and continue to explore what works best for you.

Appendix

A. Sample Fasting Plans and Protocols

Sample fasting plans and protocols vary in duration, frequency, and flexibility, allowing individuals to choose the approach that best suits their goals and lifestyle. One common fasting plan is intermittent fasting, which involves cycling between periods of eating and fasting. For instance, the 16/8 method entails fasting for 16 hours each day and consuming meals within an 8-hour window. Another popular approach is the 5:2 method, where individuals eat normally for five days a week and restrict calorie intake to about 500-600 calories on the remaining two non-consecutive days. Extended fasting protocols involve fasting for 24-48 hours or even longer on occasion. Time-restricted eating is a simpler approach, focusing on shortening the daily eating window to 10, 8, or even 6 hours. These sample fasting plans can be adapted to individual preferences and health needs, offering flexibility while still reaping the potential benefits of fasting. As with any dietary change, it's crucial to consult with a healthcare professional before embarking on a fasting plan, especially for those with specific health conditions or concerns.

B. Fasting-Friendly Recipes and Meal Ideas

Fasting-friendly recipes and meal ideas can be delicious, nutritious, and satisfying, making your fasting journey enjoyable and sustainable. Here are some options for meals that are suitable for various fasting protocols:

I. Time-Restricted Eating (e.g., 16/8):
- Breakfast: Greek yogurt with berries and a drizzle of honey, or avocado toast with a sprinkle of seeds.

- Lunch: Grilled chicken salad with mixed greens, cherry tomatoes, cucumber, and a light vinaigrette dressing.
- Dinner: Baked salmon with roasted asparagus and quinoa.

2. **Intermittent Fasting:**
   - Breakfast: Spinach and feta omelet with a side of fresh fruit.
   - Lunch: Turkey lettuce wraps with avocado and sliced bell peppers.
   - Dinner: Cauliflower rice stir-fry with tofu, broccoli, and snap peas.

3. **5:2 Fasting:**
   - On fasting days (500-600 calories):
     - Breakfast: Smoothie with spinach, almond milk, banana, and protein powder.
     - Lunch: Vegetable soup with chickpeas and a small whole-grain roll.
     - Dinner: Grilled shrimp skewers with zucchini noodles.

4. **Extended Fasting (24-48 hours):**
   - Breaking the fast:
     - Vegetable broth or bone broth for rehydration and electrolytes.

- A light meal like scrambled eggs with sautéed spinach and mushrooms.

5. **Modified Fasting:**
    - Choose fasting days based on your preferences and schedule. On fasting days, consume lighter meals with fewer calories, such as salads, soups, or smoothies.

General Tips:

- Stay hydrated with water, herbal teas, or black coffee during fasting periods.
- Incorporate nutrient-dense foods with lean proteins, healthy fats, and colorful vegetables during non-fasting periods.
- Experiment with herbs and spices to add flavor to your meals without relying on high-calorie sauces or dressings.
- Plan and prepare your meals in advance to ensure you have fasting-friendly options readily available.

Remember that fasting-friendly meals should align with your personal dietary preferences and health needs. Customize these meal ideas to suit your tastes and enjoy a variety of nutritious foods that support your fasting journey. Consult with a registered dietitian or healthcare professional for personalized advice and to ensure that your fasting approach meets your nutritional requirements.

The End.

Milton Keynes UK
Ingram Content Group UK Ltd.
UKHW021308270823
427563UK00023B/791